Aminata Tieba Traore

Evaluation of medical device sterilization processes and

Aminata Tieba Traore

Evaluation of medical device sterilization processes and

The case of seven hospitals in Mali and Senegal

ScienciaScripts

Imprint

Any brand names and product names mentioned in this book are subject to trademark, brand or patent protection and are trademarks or registered trademarks of their respective holders. The use of brand names, product names, common names, trade names, product descriptions etc. even without a particular marking in this work is in no way to be construed to mean that such names may be regarded as unrestricted in respect of trademark and brand protection legislation and could thus be used by anyone.

Cover image: www.ingimage.com

This book is a translation from the original published under ISBN 978-3-639-54719-1.

Publisher:
Sciencia Scripts
is a trademark of
Dodo Books Indian Ocean Ltd. and OmniScriptum S.R.L publishing group

120 High Road, East Finchley, London, N2 9ED, United Kingdom
Str. Armeneasca 28/1, office 1, Chisinau MD-2012, Republic of Moldova, Europe
Printed at: see last page
ISBN: 978-620-5-85304-7

Table of contents :

CHEIKH ANTA DIOP UNIVERSITY OF DAKAR

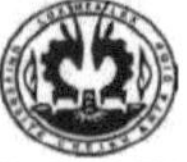

FACULTY OF MEDICINE, PHARMACY AND DENTISTRY
*****

Laboratory of Pharmacology and Pharmacodynamics
*****

EVALUATION OF STERILIZATION PROCESSES FOR MEDICAL DEVICES AND SURGICAL TEXTILES IN SEVEN HOSPITALS IN MALI AND SENEGAL

Presented by

Aminata Tièba TRAORÉ

STATE DOCTOR OF PHARMACY

Jury members

President	**M. Amadou Moctar**	**DIEYE**	**Professor**
Memory Director	**M. Bara**	**NDIAYE**	**Professor**
Member	**M. Oumar**	**THIOUNE**	**Associate Professor**
Member	**M. Djibril**	**FALL**	**Associate Professor**

Dedication:

I dedicate this work:

To Allah: I give thanks to GOD the Almighty, the Most Merciful, for giving me the strength and health to complete this work.

To my father : Tièba TRAORE

Dad, you were an example of courage, perseverance and honesty in the accomplishment of a job well done. You never failed in your duty, you remain for us an exemplary father. May God grant you a long life to see us succeed in life.

To my mother : Aminata COULIBALY

Mom, this work is the fruit of the education we received from you. May God grant you a long life and excellent health.

To my brothers and sisters:

Mariame, Kotiè, Fatoumata, Dioma, Alhousseyni, Alhassane, Zaînabou, Aîcha, Ibrahima, Family unity is priceless; we must all remain united and supportive forever.

This work is yours; find in it all my affection and my deep attachment. May this work serve as an example to you and encourage you to do better.

Acknowledgements

To all my aunts and uncles especially, **Mrs. DIAKITE Ami TRAORÉ, Niamanto DIARRA, Moussa COULIBALY and Zanafon OUATTARA**, thank you for the advice and encouragement.

To my friends and accomplices: Dr. Mariam DIAMCOUMBA DOUMBIA, Dr. Fatoumata MAIGA, Dr. Aminata O TRAORÉ, Dr. Alamako Doumbia, Dr. Khadidiatou FALL THIAM, thank you for everything.

To **Dr. Yacouba CISSOKO, Dr. Issa DIARRA and Dr. Madani MARIKO**, thank you.

To the staff of the central pharmacy and IB of the Aristide Le Dantec Hospital,

To the faculty of the FMPOS of Mali

To all my colleagues, especially to the students in the Master of Hospital and Community Pharmacy, thank you and good luck to all.

I would like to thank all the staff of the hospitals included in our study:
-   Mali (CHU-Gabriel Touré, Point-G and Kati, and the CHME)
- Senegal (Hôpital Principal de Dakar, Hôpital Aristide Le Dantec and Hôpital Général de Grand Yoff)

I thank the faculty of UCAD in Senegal, especially

To Professor **Babacar FAYE**, Coordinator of the Master of Hospital and Community Pharmacy,

To Professor **Amadou Moctar DIEYE**, for his contribution to this work,

My thanks go naturally to Professor **Elimane Mariko**, we will never forget what you have done for us. Thank you

To **Dr. Loséni BENGALY**, you helped me a lot in this work. I always ask God not to be ungrateful to you.

To the **Belgian Technical Cooperation** which allowed us to realize this work,

To all the Senegalese and Malian communities, for your sympathy. Good luck to all.

To all those who have contributed in any way to the realization of this work, thank you.

List of abbreviations

AFSSAPS : Agence Française de Sécurité Sanitaire des Produits de Santé

OMS : Organisation Mondiale de la Santé

CSP : Code de la Santé Public

PUI : Pharmacie à Usage Intérieur

ARH : Agence de Régulation Hospitalière

DM : Dispositif Médical

EN : Norme Européenne

NF : Normalisation en France

ISO : Organisation internationale de normalisation

AFNOR : Association française de normalisation

CEE : Communauté Économique Européenne

CE : Communauté Européenne

CHU-GT : Centre Hospitalo-Universitaire de Gabriel Touré.

CHU-Point-G : Centre Hospitalo-Universitaire du Point G.

CHU-Kati : Centre Hospitalo-Universitaire de Kati.

CHME : Centre Hospitalier Mère-Enfant "Luxembourg".

CHU-HALD : Hôpital Aristide Le Dantec.

HPD : Hôpital Principal de Dakar.

HOGGY : Hôpital Général de Grand Yoff.

AHR : Autorité de Réglementation Hospitalière

PUI : Pharmacie à Usage Intérieur

BPS : Bonnes Pratiques de Stérilisation.

BPPH : Bonnes pratiques de Pharmacie Hospitalière

WFHSS : Forum Mondial pour des Fournitures Stériles à l'Hôpital

% : Pourcentage

N : Nombre

US : Unité de Stérilisation

Introduction

The hospital is the ultimate care facility. However, the patient is at risk of acquiring a nosocomial infection. Sterilization plays an essential role in preventing this type of infectious risk[1] .

The risk of infection is the result of many parameters related to care. The good practice guide on the disinfection of medical devices (1998) has established a classification of devices according to the degree of invasiveness and the infectious risk in order to determine the level of treatment required. The prevention of nosocomial infections is a major objective for hospitals. The best possible quality of care must be provided. The use of single-use equipment improves patient comfort and represents a guarantee of quality and health safety. However, some medical devices cannot be used as single-use for cost reasons and benefit from this industrial approach (surgical instruments, endoscopes)[2] .

Nowadays, there is a growing awareness for safety during care and for the prevention of healthcare associated infections. This is reflected in the implementation of the first global challenge for patient safety: "Clean care is safer care". Sterilization of medical devices and surgical drapes plays a major role in quality assurance of care. It is one of the fundamental elements of the various measures to prevent healthcare associated infections. Sterilization in hospitals is a pharmaceutical activity whose objective is to deliver sterile products to practitioners. According to the Good Hospital Pharmacy Practices[2] adequate treatment of medical devices requires sufficient human, material and financial resources[3] . In developing countries such as Mali or Senegal, the organization of sterilization in hospitals has not reached the desired level of standards. In fact, sterilization procedures are often not centralized at the level of a department, and the staff in charge of sterilization have rarely received specific training on this subject and are not sufficiently aware of the limits of the techniques used. Systematic control is not always carried out. Add to this the inadequacy of the architecture of the premises, which does not meet the specified requirements for sterilization of medical devices.

Our study aims to evaluate the Good Sterilization Practices (G.S.P.) in relation to the Standards in hospitals in Mali and Senegal. It will allow us to formulate recommendations to improve sterilization processes.

This work is part of the Master's program in Hospital and Community Pharmacy at Cheick Anta Diop University in Dakar.

In the study, we present the problem of the sterilization of medical devices and operating fields at the level of hospitals and we formulate proposals for the reorganization of the field at the level of the studied structures.

In the hospital environment, the pharmacist is responsible for the quality of sterilized materials. He must ensure it. Several methods are possible, we have chosen one of them:

I. PART ONE: GENERAL

11.1 SOME DEFINITIONS :

> ### Sterility

According to the European Pharmacopoeia, sterility is defined as the absence of viable micro-organisms [2].

The sterility of all items in a sterilization population cannot be absolutely guaranteed or verified. There is always a certain statistical probability that a micro-organism can survive sterilization[4] .

Sterility is generally considered an absolute concept. However, it is the probability of having one non-sterile unit in a million sterilized units. There is therefore a very low probability that a microbe survives after sterilization, regardless of the effectiveness of the methods and means implemented. In practice, it is impossible to sterilize at 100%. In other words, sterilization is an operation to reduce contamination, with a maximum threshold of one millionth.

Sterility is the relative absence of pathogenic and saprophytic germs or the absence of any microorganisms in vegetative form, spores, pathogenic or not.

> ### Sterile

The European standard EN 556[6] defines sterile as the state of a medical device that is free of viable microorganisms. Due to the nature of microbial inactivation kinetics, it is not possible to verify that every device, taken at random from a population of sterilized devices, meets the definition. In order for a medical device to be labeled "sterile", the theoretical probability of a viable microorganism being present on that device must be equal to or less than $1/10^6$ [4] .

> ### Sterilization

Sterilization is the "implementation of a set of methods and means aimed at eliminating all living micro-organisms, of whatever nature, carried by a perfectly cleaned object"[8] . Sterilization is a process or a set of operations, therefore a process. This process should not be confused with the result: sterility[1] .

Steam sterilization is the reference process at the hospital[7] .

> ### Medical devices (DM)

According to the Medical Devices Directive 93/42/EEC, a MD is an instrument, apparatus, equipment or software intended by its manufacturer to be used in humans for the purpose of, inter alia, diagnosis, prevention, control, treatment, mitigation of disease or injury [10].

The main action of a medical device is not obtained by pharmacological or immunological means or by metabolism, it is essentially mechanical.

Medical devices are classified into four classes according to their level of danger. The marketing of medical devices is carried out under the responsibility of their manufacturers after they have affixed the CE mark, which attests to their compliance with the essential health and safety requirements set by the European directives. The AFSSAPS, like the other authorities in charge of these devices, intervenes, a posteriori, to monitor the market, i.e. to ensure the conformity with the health and safety requirements of the devices placed on the market on the national territory [10]

> **Sterilization cycle of reusable DM:**

The sterilization cycle is defined as the automatic sequences of operations carried out in a sterilizer with the aim of reaching the sterile state.

> **Sterilizer**

Apparatus used to sterilize surgical equipment, dressings and injectable drugs[11] .

> **Packaging: protection of the sterile state**

The sterile state, obtained after the sterilization operation, is preserved thanks to the packaging which must fulfill several functions until the moment of use of the sterile article. The packaging must be permeable to the sterilizing agent. It constitutes an impenetrable barrier to microorganisms, protects the material while allowing its extraction and use under aseptic conditions.

> **Bowie-Dick test**

This is a test to be done at the beginning of the day, before using the sterilizer and at least once every 24 hours. This test verifies the rapid and complete penetration of steam into a porous load and the elimination of air (thus indirectly the operation of the vacuum circuit). Ready-to-use Bowie-Dick test packs or an electronic device are preferably used for this purpose. The test pack is placed alone in the tank of the heated device and the test cycle, which includes a pre-treatment and a plateau at 134°C / 3.5 min, is started[5] .

11.2 FRENCH AND EUROPEAN REGULATIONS AND RECOMMENDATIONS ON STERILIZATION

This regulation is based on certain texts of which :

Law n° 91748 of July 31, 1991 on hospital reform, dealing in particular with : The organization of hospital structures, of which articles L 713.5 to 11 are related to hospital unions.

The Decree n° 2004-451 of May 21, 2004 relating to the internal use pharmacy which is a document attesting to the adoption of the system to be established when there is subcontracting between care structures in the context of sterilization. Indeed, the ordinary Law 2004-806 of August 9, 2004 relating to public health policy significantly modifies article L. 5126-2 of the CSP allowing the PUI "to ensure all or part of the sterilization of medical devices on behalf of another establishment.

Article L 5126-5 modified by the law N° 2002-73 of January 17, 2002 of social modernization (JO 15 of 18/01/02)

The internal use pharmacy is notably responsible for: ensuring, in compliance with the rules governing the operation of the establishment, the management, supply, preparation, control, holding and dispensing of medicines, products or objects mentioned in article L 4211-1, as well as sterile medical devices and ensuring their quality.

Order n° 2003-850 of September 4, 2003 simplifying the organization and functioning of the health system (J.O. of September 6, 2003)

The director of the ARH may authorize an IUP to carry out sterilization of medical devices on behalf of another establishment. This article is also completed in order to allow the PUI of a health cooperation grouping to provide sterilization for another establishment[12] .

NB: There is no regulatory text for sterilization in Mali and Senegal.

11.3 DIFFERENT STAGES OF STERILIZATION

A preliminary provision to the sterilization is to be noted **"One sterilizes well only what is clean"** the various stages of the sterilization are illustrated by the following figure

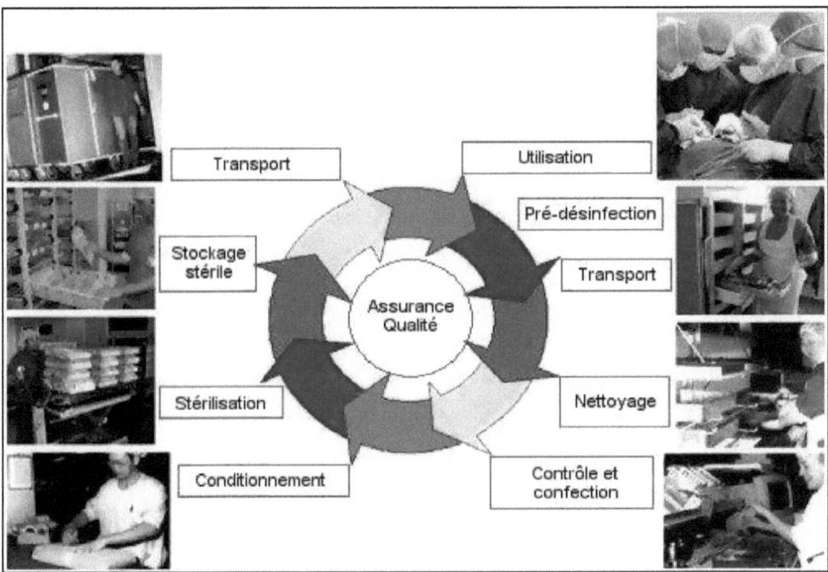

Figure No. 1: Steps of sterilization [13]

11.3.1 Pre-disinfection

Pre-disinfection or pre-treatment is the first operation to be performed on soiled DM in order to reduce the population of micro-organisms and to facilitate subsequent cleaning.

Pre-disinfection is also intended to protect personnel and avoid environmental contamination.

Pre-disinfection is performed in the operating room by immersion in a detergent and bactericidal solution. The product must comply with the standards, NF EN 1040[9] , NF EN 13727[14] and NF EN 13624[15] . These properties give it an activity on germs (bactericide, virucide and fungicide)[16] .

11.3.2 Receiving and sorting:

When the dirty devices arrive in the sterilization department, it is necessary to check that the pre-disinfection steps have been carried out effectively, that the instruments have been identified on the accompanying slip, in order to organize their subsequent handling according to the suppliers' recommendations, that there is a possible risk situation (Prion) requiring the implementation of a specific procedure, and the general condition of the device. This initial sorting should make it possible to set aside deteriorated instruments and choose the cleaning method best suited to each device. If this information is not available, the sterilization department cannot take charge of the devices and the agent in charge of receiving them must refer the matter to his or her supervisor[16] .

11.3.3 Cleaning:

The cleaning aims to obtain the minimum level of contamination and has for objectives to eliminate dirt, especially organic matter and to prevent the formation of a bio-film[34] . Cleaning also includes:

Rinsing: the purpose of rinsing is to remove detergent residues from the instruments

Drying: The purpose of drying is to remove water and residual moisture from the instruments.

Sorting and checking: in order to sterilize only functional medical devices and articles that are fit for purpose, individual checks are necessary to verify the general condition of the material:

- absence of stains, deformations, traces of corrosion for the instruments,

- functionality of instruments, e.g. articulated (pliers), cutting (scissors), gripping (needle holder), if applicable, absence of stains, tears, holes, foreign particles for textile articles

11.3.4 Packaging:

Packaging is an essential step in the sterilization process. The integrity of the packaging allows the sterile state to be maintained until use. Packaging must be carried out as soon as possible after washing to avoid any possible re-contamination. It is carried out on dry instruments in good condition. The checking of the instruments must follow a precise procedure and must be carried out by trained personnel

- **Types of packaging**

The different types of packaging are :

- single-use packaging such as crepe or non-woven paper, bags and sleeves,

- reusable packaging such as centenarians.

The label on the package contributes to traceability.

ƒ During sterilization :

The packaging allows the passage of the sterilizing agent.

ƒ After sterilization :

The packaging prevents the passage of micro-organisms and maintains the sterile state until use.[16] .

Means of protection of the personnel :

In packaging areas, wrist and hand jewelry promote the persistence of transient flora by creating ecological niches that are not easily accessible to hand washing.

It has been proven that the presence of a ring is a factor that favors the germ, the presence of bacteria of the transient flora on the hands whatever the shape of the ring: thick, tight, thin or other. This dirt is poorly eliminated when washing or disinfecting the hands. The skin under the rings is not easily accessible to hand hygiene procedures. The wedding ring is only a special case of a ring. Sterilization staff should remove all rings, including the wedding band, watch, and bracelets, before beginning work.

According to the BPPH, the nails must be cut short. Nail polish is forbidden because by chipping, it creates small cavities that become ecological niches. Artificial nails are forbidden: it is proven that dirt and microorganisms slip between the artificial nail and the natural nail.

Agents should be aware that these instructions are intended to protect them and their surroundings as well as the medical devices

11.3.5 Labeling

Labeling identifies the device and contributes to the traceability of the treatment.

It must mention the name of the device and the expiration date.

Information about the sterilization cycle (date, batch number) can be accessed in the form of a barcode.

Each package has a physico-chemical indicator of passage to verify that the device has been subjected to a sterilization cycle[16] .

11.3.6 Storage

It is intended to maintain the integrity of the packaging of sterile medical devices for a specific period of time.

> labelled packages stored in a dedicated, regularly maintained arsenal,

> away from heat, humidity and direct daylight (ultraviolet radiation),

> storage to facilitate stock rotation,

> no crushed packages or folded pouches to avoid compromising the sterile state **[16]**.

11.3.7 The sterilization process:

According to the definition given in the H.P.P.G., a "process or procedure is a set of related means and activities that transforms inputs into outputs. These means may include personnel, finances, facilities, equipment, techniques and methods."

According to ISO 9000, a process is a set of interrelated or interactive activities that transforms inputs into outputs.

The processes can be classified into 3 categories.

A process is defined by characteristics:

* concept of an owner
* its objectives
* its customers and suppliers

* the actors allowing its realization
* its input and output data
* the methods allowing its implementation: documentary system the means to implement it.

It is controlled and monitored through steering indicators and other evaluation methods, including audits[17] .

11.3.8 The quality

According to the B.P.P.H., quality is "the set of characteristics of an entity that gives it the ability to satisfy expressed and implicit needs".

Thus, in the context of the sterilization activity, quality can be defined as the confidence of the health care staff that they have the right sterile product for the right patient at the right time[17] .

11.3.9 Quality Assurance

Each step in a sterilization cycle is critical to the proper use and safety of a sterile instrument or other device during a medical procedure. A mistake or failure at any step can cause re-contamination that renders the entire procedure useless. This can result in significant additional costs and serious damage, as well as endangering the lives of patients and staff. That is why each step will be subject to strict monitoring. This is achieved by a Quality Assurance System, in which each step of the sterilization cycle is analyzed, documented and monitored, as a true tool to control a sterile product, safe for patients and users, efficient, which meets predefined quality standards, and for an acceptable price[13] .

II.   PART TWO: EXPERIMENTAL WORK

I: CONTEXT OF THE STUDY

We conducted this survey in a context generally marked by the non-existence of data relating to the practice of sterilization in hospitals in Mali and Senegal, with the exception of a survey on the sterilization of surgical DM carried out in 2010 in seven hospitals in the Dakar region by DIOUF WC[18]. The audit team's motivations were in line with the overall improvement of care to which these establishments have subscribed.

II: OBJECTIVES OF THE STUDY

11.1   GENERAL OBJECTIVE

The general objective of this work is to evaluate the practice of the sterilization process of reusable medical devices (M.D.) and surgical textiles in seven hospitals located in Mali and Senegal in comparison with the recommendations and regulations in force.

11.2   SPECIFIC OBJECTIVES

- Describe the architectural design of the selected sterilization units.
- Evaluate the steps of the sterilization process in each selected sterilization unit in relation to current standards.
- Determine whether or not a quality assurance system exists.
- Evaluate the profile of the personnel employed in the selected sterilization units.
- Suggest areas for improvement to correct any malfunctions noted.

111.1 Framework of the study

The study was conducted in the sterilization units of four hospitals in Mali and three in Senegal.

The institutions involved in the study are:

> **For Mali :**

The Gabriel Touré University Hospital Center (CHU-GT)

The University Hospital Center of Point G (CHU-Point-G)

The University Hospital of Kati (CHU-Kati)

The Mother and Child Hospital Center "Luxembourg" (CHME)

> **For Senegal :**

The Aristide Le Dantec University Hospital (HALD)

The Army Training Hospital (Hôpital Principal de Dakar (HPD))

Grand Yoff General Hospital (HOGGY)

In Mali, there were 32 care units with 1033 hospital beds. One thousand five hundred and sixty nine (1569) healthcare professionals and administrators worked in the hospital. The total number of patients admitted in 2009 was thirty two thousand two hundred and forty six (32286).

In Senegal, there were 43 intensive care units with 1049 hospital beds. Two thousand one hundred and eighty nine (2189) nursing and administrative professionals were employed and the number of patients admitted to the hospital was 34796 with a total hospitalization day of 245127.

Observations were made in the sterilization units and in the operating rooms.

111.2 . Materials and methods

For the purposes of our study, we used:

Guidelines such as the Guide for the care of medical devices in sterilization, recommendations for the manual processing of non-autoclavable and autoclavable medical devices, etc. An evaluation grid developed from the guidelines.

111.2.1. Type of study

We conducted a descriptive study in the sterilization process. [Appendix 1].

111.2.2. Study period

The survey was conducted over a four-month period, with two months in each country (in Mali from September 15 to November 15, 2012 and in Senegal from December 1, 2011 to January 31, 2012).

111.2.3. Study sample

Our work was a descriptive study of the sterilization process in hospitals. It focused on the personnel present in the sterilization units; reusable medical devices and surgical textiles in four hospitals in Mali and three in Senegal.

We have focused in particular on the different operations of the sterilization process in the sterilization units

III.2.4. Choice of **III.2.4. Choice of evaluation criteria**

This choice was based on the normative regulations, recommendations and guidelines for sterilization (NF EN).

- **Inclusion criteria**
- Third referral hospitals
- Locate in Mali and Senegal
- Have a centralized sterilization unit
- Hospital agreement to participate in the study
- **Non-inclusion criterion:**

Third referral hospitals in Mali and Senegal without a centralized unit.

Third referral hospitals located outside Mali and Senegal.

111.2.5. Study Materials:

Developed questionnaires,

Logbook used to monitor the sterilization cycle,

Record of inputs used for sterilization,

Register of materials to be sterilized at the level of the care services

Observation sheet for sterilization techniques

111.2.6. Development of survey forms:

- The first part involved surveys of personnel involved in sterilization activities.

The second part dealt with the direct observation from the collection of soiled DM to the sterilization following all the steps of the BPS process.

111.2.7. Choice of theme

The choice of the theme started from a personal observation during my practical training, justified by the existence of dysfunctions noted in the application of the directives and recommendations of the sterilization process.

111.2.8. Data Collection Method:

The data were collected through a questionnaire (Appendix N°1) on the steps of good sterilization practice in the hospital. To do this, different steps were developed:

> Interviews with the managers of the sterilization unit
> The use of an open and closed-ended questionnaire;
> Direct observation of sterilization operations in the sterilization unit and the operating room;

111.2.9. Information sources

They are made up, on the one hand, of the supervisors of the services concerned, whose answers made it possible to fill in the evaluation grids and, on the other hand, of our observation of the sterilization procedure.

111.2.10. Data collection

The data were collected by interviewing the supervisors of the sterilization units concerned and by observation of the practices. For the purposes of observation, we spent 32 days in the operating rooms of the departments concerned, two days a week.

111.2.11. Data processing

Data were entered and analyzed using Excel version 2007, EPI 3.3.2 info 2005. The frequencies of "Yes" and "No" were calculated according to the following formulas:

$$\text{Frequency of Yes} = x \; \frac{\text{Total number of "Yes" votes}}{\text{Total number of "Yes" + Total number of "No}} \; 100$$

$$\text{Frequency of No} = x \; \frac{\text{Total number of "No" votes}}{\text{Total number of Yes + Total number of No}} \; 100$$

111.2.12. ANALYSIS OF RESULTS

The analysis and discussion of the results consisted of identifying the "*strong points*" (*SP*) and the "*weak points*" (*WP*). A result is qualified as a "*Strong Point*" when the total of "*Yes*" for the criterion concerned is at least equal to 3 out of 4 (3/4) for Mali and 2 out of 3 (2/3) for Senegal. Any criterion for which the total of "*No*" *is* equal to (3/4) for Mali and (2/3) for Senegal is considered a *weak point.*

Frequency of Yes: results meeting current standards

Frequency of No: results that do not comply with current standards

IV.1 Architectural design

Table II: Distribution of sterilization units according to the supervisory department in the different study sites in the two countries

In Mali

Sterilization service of the guardianship	Frequency (n)	%
Pharmacy	0	0
Operating room	4	100
Totals	**4**	**100**

(n= number of hospitals, in Mali = 4, in Senegal =3, total n = 7)

In Mali, no sterilization unit met the standards of the BPS (being attached to the pharmacy).

In Senegal

Sterilization service of the guardianship	Frequency (n)	%
Pharmacy	1	33
Operating room	3	67
Totals	**3**	**100**

(n= number of hospitals, in Mali = 4, in Senegal =3, total n = 7)

In Senegal, only one hospital met GHP standards

Table III: Architectural design and BPS compliance

Standards	Mali		Senegal		Total for the 2 countries	
	Yes	No	Yes	No	Yes	No
Existence of 3 separate production areas (dirty, clean and sterile)	0	4	1	2	1	6
Design of the premises allows to respect the "principle of the forward march".	0	4	1	2	1	6
Existence of areas dedicated to hand hygiene (water points, hydroalcoholic solution dispensers)	0	4	1	2	1	6
Existence of suitable areas for the storage of consumables)	0	4	1	2	1	6
Existence of a checkroom	0	4	1	2	1	6
U S located in the building housing the block	4	0	2	1	6	1

	Mali Yes	Mali No	Senegal Yes	Senegal No	The 2 country Yes	The 2 country No
Area estimated to be sufficient	0	4	1	2	1	6
Are the production areas easy to access? clean	1	3	1	2	2	5
Does the sterile material circuit avoid re-contamination	0	4	1	2	1	6
Percentage	**14%**	**86%**	**37%**	**63%**	**24%**	**76%**

(n= number of hospitals, in Mali = 4, in Senegal =3, total n = 7)

In both countries the compliance of the architectural design and the respect of the BPS was 24%, this rate was lower in Mali with 14%.

IV.2 The steps of the sterilization process :

IV.2.1 Pre-disinfection and cleaning

Table IV: Distribution of compliance of processes used for pre-disinfection and cleaning

Standards	Mali Yes	Mali No	Senegal Yes	Senegal No	The 2 countr Yes	countr y No
Products in accordance with the standards in force	2	2	1	2	3	4
Soaking of the DMs immediately after the intervention	2	2	1	2	3	4
DM transported in closed containers	2	2	1	2	3	4
DM transported in transport cabinets	0	4	0	3	0	7
Machine cleaning (washing machine)	0	4	2	1	2	5
Manual washing	4	0	3	0	7	0
Daily cleaning of production areas	2	2	2	1	4	3
Percentage	**43%**	**58%**	**48%**	**52%**	**45%**	**55%**

(n= number of hospitals, in Mali = 4, in Senegal =3, total n = 7)

In both countries, the standards of the pre-disinfection and cleaning processes were respected in 45% of the cases, this rate being relatively higher in Senegal (48%)

IV.2.2 Secondary packaging practice

(n= number of hospitals, in Mali = 4, in Senegal =3, total n = 7)

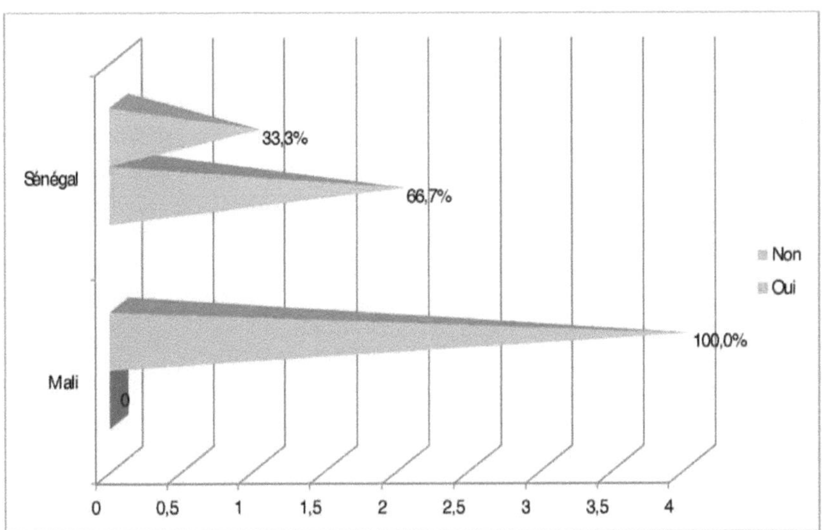

Figure N°2 : Distribution of secondary packaging use by country

In Mali, none of the sterilization units used secondary packaging of medical devices and surgical textiles, but this was a relatively common practice in Senegal (66.7%).

(n= number of hospitals, in Mali = 4, in Senegal =3, total n = 7)

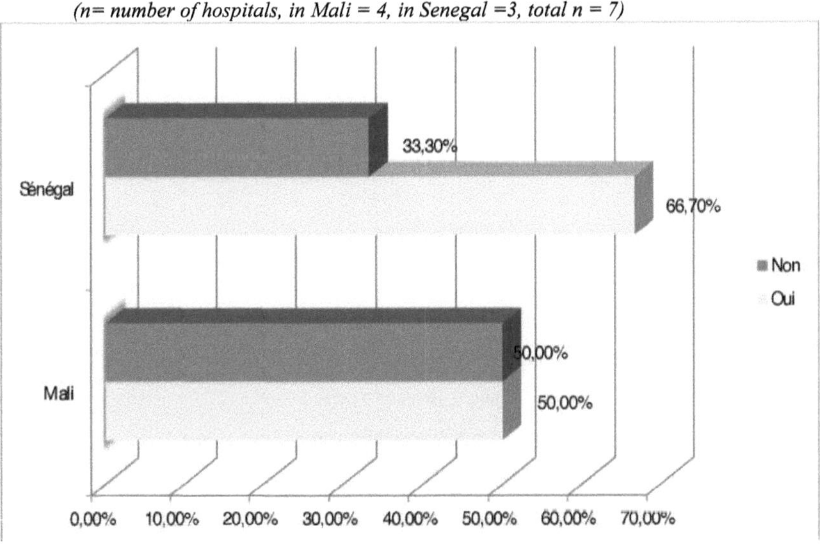

Figure N°3 : Distribution of autoclaves for the sterilization of metallic DM The sterilization of metallic DM with steam was 50% in Mali against 67% in Senegal.

IV.2.4 Different sterilization trays (or sterilization cycles) used on metallic DM, plastic DM and surgical textiles.

Table V: Distribution of the sterilization tray for metallic DM, plastic DM and surgical textiles

Standards	Mali		Senegal		The 2 countries	
	Yes	No	Yes	No	Yes	No
134° for 18min metallic DM	*0*	*4*	*1*	*2*	*1*	*5*
134° for 10 min textiles	1	3	1	1	2	5
125° for 20 min DM plastics	0	4	1	1	1	6
180° for 60 min DM metal (poupinel)	0	4	0	3	0	7
Percentage	6 %	94%	30%	70%	15%	85%

(n= number of hospitals, in Mali = 4, in Senegal =3, total n = 7)

In both countries, compliance with the sterilization tray for metal, plastic and surgical textiles was 15%. This practice was almost non-existent in Mali (6%) compared to 30% in Senegal.

Table VII: Distribution of steam sterilizer (Autoclave) qualification at installation and re-qualification within the required timeframe (every 18 months).

	Mali		Senegal		The 2 countries	
Standards	Yes	No	Yes	No	Yes	No
Qualification of sterilizers at installation	4	0	3	0	7	0
Requalification of steam sterilizers within the required timeframe (18 months)	0	4	1	2	1	6
Percentage	50	50%	67	33	57	43

(n= number of hospitals, in Mali = 4, in Senegal =3, total n = 7)

All the autoclaves were qualified at the time of installation, only one sterilization unit in Senegal was re-qualifying these autoclaves within the required 18-month period.

Table VIII: Distribution of reusable DMs that have been labeled.

	Mali		Senegal		The 2 countries	
Standards	Yes	No	Yes	No	Yes	No
Batch number for the load	0	4	1	2	1	6
Date of sterilization	0	4	1	2	1	6
Use by date	0	4	1	2	1	6
Sterilization cycle (e.g. FLASH or ATNC cycle)	0	4	1	2	1	6

	Mali Yes	Mali No	Senegal Yes	Senegal No	The 2 countries Yes	The 2 countries No
Identification of sterilized material	**4**	0	**1**	2	**1**	6
Name of the operator	**0**	4	**1**	2	**1**	6
Is there a tracking sheet for the material to be sterilized	**0**	4	**1**	2	**1**	6
Is the traceability of sterilized DM carried out?	**0**	4	**1**	2	**1**	6
Management of non-conformities	**0**	4	**1**	2	**1**	6
Percentage	**11%**	**89 %**	**33%**	**67 %**	**14%**	**86 %**

(n= number of hospitals, in Mali = 4, in Senegal =3, total n = 7)

In both countries, according to BPS standards, only 14% of the facilities labelled their MDs and surgical textiles, 11% in Mali and 33% in Senegal.

Table IX: Distribution of the different methods of storage of MDs and operating textiles

	Mali Yes	Mali No	Senegal Yes	Senegal No	The 2 countries Yes	The 2 countries No
Standards						
FIFO system (1er in, 1er out) implemented	0	4		12	1	6
Storage equipment avoids any overcrowding	0	4		12	1	6
Favourable storage room (protected from light), moisture and contaminations of all kinds. natures)	0	4		12	1	6
Delivery	0	4		12	1	6
Percentage	**0**	**100%**	**33%**	**67%**	**14%**	**86%**

(n= number of hospitals, in Mali = 4, in Senegal =3, total n = 7)

Only in Senegal (33%) were the storage of medical devices and textiles respected.

IV.2.5 Equipment available in the sterilization units

Table VI: Distribution of equipment available for sterilization

Standards	Mali Yes	Mali No	Senegal Yes	Senegal No	The 2 countries Yes	The 2 countries No
Drainer	**0**	4	**0**	3	**7**	0
Washbasin	**0**	4	**1**	2	**1**	6
Sink	**4**	0	**2**	1	**1**	6
Washing cabin	**0**	4	**1**	2	**6**	1
Washing machine	**0**	4	**2**	1	**5**	2

	Mali Yes	Mali No	Senegal Yes	Senegal No	The 2 countries Yes	The 2 countries No
Heat sealer	1	3	2	1	3	4
Ribbon with passage indicator	2	2	2	1	4	3
Bags or sleeves	1	3	2	1	3	4
containers	2	2	3	0	5	2
Hydro-alcoholic solution dispenser	0	4	1	2	1	6
An autoclave available	4	0	2	1	6	1
Two autoclaves available	0	4	0	0	0	7
Three autoclaves available	0	4	1	2	1	6
A doll available	2	0	2	1	4	3
Two dolls available	1	3	0	3	1	3
No dolls available	1	3	1	2	2	5
Percentage	**29%**	**71%**	**49%**	**51%**	**46%**	**54%**

(n= number of hospitals, in Mali = 4, in Senegal =3, total n = 7)

IV.3. Quality assurance

In Senegal, 49% of the equipment was available for sterilization compared to 29% in Mali.

IV.3. Quality assurance

Table VII: Existence of a quality assurance system

	Mali Yes	Mali No	Senegal Yes	Senegal No	The 2 countries Or	The 2 countries No
Standards						
Existence of a quality policy	0	4	0	3	0	7
Operating organization chart (definition responsibilities)	0	4	0	3	0	7
Organization described by means of procedures	0	4	0	3	0	7
Recordings	0	4	0	3	0	7
Percentage	**0**	**100%**	**0**	**100%**	**0**	**100%**

(n= number of hospitals, in Mali = 4, in Senegal =3, total n = 7)

The quality assurance system was non-existent in both countries.

IV.5 Personnel identification (human resources) :

Table X: Compliance with standards in terms of qualification of personnel involved in sterilization, according to the different study sites

Standards	Mali Yes	Mali No	Senegal Yes	Senegal No	The 2 country Yes	The 2 country No
Head of US is a pharmacist	0	4	1	2	1	6
Head of US is a physician	4	4	2	1	6	1
Staff trained in relation to the standard	0	4	1	2	1	6
Staff with continuing education	0	4	1	2	1	6
PIAS, senior health technicians	3	1	1	2	4	3

PIAS, Pharmacy Preparers	1	3	1	2	2	5
PIAS, medical assistants	2	2	1	2	3	4
PIAS, instrumentalists	0	4	2	1	2	5
PIAS, Caregivers	1	3	2	1	3	4
PIAS, maneuvers	3	1	1	2	4	3
PIAS, volunteers	2	2	0	3	2	5
Percentage	**33 %**	**67 %**	**39%**	**61 %**	**38%**	**62 %**

(n= number of hospitals, in Mali = 4, in Senegal =3, total n = 7)

* *PIAS: Personnel Involved in Sterilization Activities*

Only one pharmacist was head of the sterilization unit, and the laborers and orderlies were more involved in sterilization activities than other health care managers.

Table XI: Distribution of personnel by means of protection by study site.

	Mali		Senegal		The 2 countries	
Standards	**Yes**	**No**	**Yes**	**No**	**Yes**	**No**
Staff vaccinated against hepatitis B	0	4	0	3	0	7
Staff underwent an intradermal test with tuberculin	n	4	n	<2	n	7
Staff benefit from medical follow-up	0	4	2	1	2	5
Staff with ordinary gloves	4	0	3	0	7	0
Staff with long machete gloves	1	3	1	2	2	5
Personnel with protective eyewear	0	4	1	2	1	6
Staff with aprons	0	4	1	2	1	6
Personnel with protective masks	0	4	1	2	1	6
Staff with overshoes	0	4	1	2	1	6
Staff with single-use tunic and pants	0	4	1	2	1	6
Percentage	**12%**	**88%**	**37%**	**63%**	**23%**	**77%**

(n= number of hospitals, in Mali = 4, in Senegal =3, total n = 7)

In both countries, 23% of the staff used the means of protection according to the standards in force; this rate was relatively low in Mali (12%)

Table XII: Results of observation of practices related to the sterilization process in hospitals in Mali and Senegal.

		Mali	Senegal
Activities	**Observations**	**Frequencies**	**Frequencies**

Pre-disinfection	preparation of the pre-treatment solution in accordance with the standards	0	1/3
	Compliant product mixed with bleach	2/4	1/3
	Bleach mixed with regular soap	2/4	0
	Ord soap alone	0	1/3
	DM packed in fields	2/4	2/3
	Respect of the soaking time at least 15 minutes	4/4	2/3
	Immediate soaking in the OR after surgery	1/4	1/3
Cleaning	Cleaning with washing machine	0	2/3
	Generally manual with brush	4/4	3/3
packaging	Production of the secondary packaging	0	1/3
	Wearing a mask in the packaging area	0	1/3
sterilization	134° for 8min metallic DM	1/4	0
	134° for 5min metallic DM	1/4	0
	Plastic DM sterilized by soaking the pre-disinfection solution	3/4	1/3

(n= number of hospitals, in Mali = 4, in Senegal =3, total n = 7)

V . DISCUSSION

V .1. Our methodology

This study was conducted to evaluate the sterilization processes in hospitals in two countries with limited resources (Mali and Senegal). Within this framework, we chose four hospitals in Mali (GabrielTOURE University Hospital Center; Point G University Hospital Center; Kati University Hospital Center and Mother and Child Hospital Center Luxembourg) and three hospitals in Senegal (Aristide Le Dantec University Hospital Center; Grand Yoff General Hospital and Dakar Main Hospital). The study was conducted with the aim of improving the quality of sterilization products, especially since poor sterilization is an important risk factor for nosocomial infections.

To our knowledge, only one study in this area has been conducted in Senegal in the Dakar region (DIOUF. WC), while in Mali, no study has addressed this subject. To better understand the problems related to sterilization, we conducted this study in a multicenter approach by including some hospitals in Mali.

This approach allowed us to describe the existing sterilization practices in each country and to compare them with the AFNOR standards for sterilization. We were thus able to measure the gaps between the practice in these units and the requirements in terms of quality. However, we were not able to establish the consequences of the shortcomings noted in the sterilization units on the quality of the products resulting from this sterilization, as our study did not include microbiological analyses performed on the products from the sterilization units evaluated.

V .2 Architectural design :

In Mali, no sterilization unit was attached to the in-house pharmacy in accordance with current standards. However, in Senegal, only one sterilization unit in the main hospital in Dakar was attached to the in-house pharmacy. The fact that the sterilization unit is not attached to the in-house pharmacy in most of the hospitals surveyed may result in poor input management. It should be remembered that the pharmacist, by virtue of his or her training, has the necessary skills to manage the <u>supply circuit of inputs usable in the hospital, including</u> sterilization <u>inputs.</u> Poor management of inputs could lead to stock shortages, resulting in a stoppage of the sterilization chain or the use of products not recommended by the standards, all of which would lead to defective sterilization.

Our results show that all the hospitals visited have a central sterilization unit. However, we found that in addition to the CSSDs, there are other sites for the sterilization of reusable medical devices in the hospitals visited. This situation leads us to believe that the central character of a sterilization unit is linked to the fact that it exclusively treats medical devices from the operating rooms. The centralization of the sterilization process should respond to the need to group all the activities concerned within the same establishment in order to obtain homogeneity and reproducibility in the treatment of medical devices[23] .

The architecture of the CSSD premises must allow, whenever possible, the respect of the principle of forward movement[28] , i.e. to go from the dirtiest to the cleanest, to reduce as much as possible the risks of contamination and confusion. The medical devices (M.D.) will therefore follow a sterilization circuit with no possibility of going backwards.

In addition, the possibility of expanding the activity must be taken into account.

According to the Good Sterilization Practices (G.S.P.)[28] and Good Hospital Pharmacy Practices (GHPP)[1] , there are different zones within the sterilization department: the washing zone, the packaging zone and the sterile output zone. Each of these areas can be structured in different elements but they will allow to follow the evolution of a MD during the sterilization, the principle being to make it progress from "contaminated" to "sterile conditioned".

One of the contributions of this work could be to contribute to the improvement of the sterilization environment, while respecting the principle of forward movement and ensuring traceability of the M.D. and surgical textiles to be sterilized.

In order to respect the "forward motion" and to maintain the Iso 8 class in the packaging area, it is judicious that the washer-disinfectors constitute a technical wall between the washing area and the packaging area. Of course, in this design, the washers have double doors with the loading door on the washing side and the unloading door on the packaging side. In our study, the Hôpital Principal de Dakar was the only hospital to have a washer that respected this wall and to practice the forward circuit. In his study on sterilization practices for medical devices in hospitals in the Dakar Region in 2010, DIOUF. W.C.[18] also made the same observation. On the other hand, a study conducted in the United Kingdom in 2007-2008 by SHAH. R et al. on cross-infection in dentistry showed that 97% of the departments surveyed had separate "dirty" and "clean" washing areas[19] . The 2007 study by BAGG. J et al. on the pre-disinfection and cleaning of reusable instruments in general dental practice, showed that 69% of the wash areas and packaging areas were not clearly defined[21] . The absence of this wall in most of the facilities involved in our study may result in the recontamination of already sterilized M.D.s. This situation could increase the rate of nosocomial infection due to the use of M.D. supposedly sterile when they are not.

It is therefore necessary to install this wall in all sterilization units in accordance with the standards in force.

It would be even better to be able to carry out a continuous quality control of the products resulting from the sterilization in order to have a guarantee of their sterility and to avoid their incrimination in nosocomial infections.

V.3 Sterilization process step :

V.3.1. Pre-disinfection

Pre-disinfection is the first treatment to be carried out on objects and materials soiled by organic matter in order to reduce their population of micro-organisms and to facilitate their subsequent cleaning.

Pre-disinfection is also intended to protect the staff when handling the instruments. It also prevents contamination of the environment. The product used should not be a protein fixative itself.

Pre-disinfection of the M.D.s was carried out immediately after the operation in the operating room at three hospitals in both countries (2/4 hospitals in Mali and 1/3 in Senegal). The other hospitals packaged the MDs in surgical textiles for transport from the operating room to the sterilization unit, and it was the sterilization unit that pre-disinfected the MDs. W.C. found that 6/7 hospitals (85.70%) performed pre-disinfection (immediate soaking) of the MDs after surgery in the operating room. The other hospitals packed the M.D.s in surgical textiles for transport from the operating room to the sterilization unit, and the sterilization unit then proceeded to pre-disinfect these M.D.s at their level. W.C.[18] , in the Dakar Region in 2010, found that 5/7 hospitals (71.4%) transported soiled MDs in surgical textiles from the operating room to the sterilization unit.

The absence of immediate pre-disinfection in the operating room can promote the development of prions and the coagulation of biological fluids on the M.D. In addition, the transport of M.D. to other premises for pre-disinfection increases the risk of accidental exposure to soiled M.D. of the personnel and the hospital environment.

The equipment of operating rooms with materials and inputs for pre-disinfection as well as the training of personnel in their use is therefore a necessity in most of the facilities we evaluated.

V.3.2. Cleaning or washing

This is the first step in the preparation of medical devices, following pre-disinfection. However, washing with a brush, which must be preceded by pre-disinfection, was carried out in the opposite direction; the medical devices were washed before being soaked in almost all of the facilities evaluated, except for the Hôpital Principal de Dakar.

According to the **NF EN ISO 15 883-2** standard, manual cleaning is no longer recommended, whereas our survey showed that the majority of sterilization units carry out manual cleaning using brushes. Indeed, manual cleaning is a risky task for the staff. In addition, we observed that outside of the Hôpital Principal de Dakar, staff do not use the recommended protective equipment for this operation, such as long-sleeved gloves, protective aprons, goggles, masks, and clogs. **BAGG. J** et **al**, in their **2007** study of pre-disinfection and cleaning of reusable instruments in general dental practice found that only 7% of staff used dry suits, 51% did not use goggles, and 57% did not use protective masks[21] . Another cross-infection control study conducted by **SHAH. R** et **al. in 2007 in the United Kingdom** found that 98% of staff had protective equipment [19].

Sterilization is a specific job, the protection of the personnel is a duty for the hospital and the head of the department must ensure that the rules for wearing work clothes are respected according to the production areas. The hospital must provide appropriate inputs and materials for sterilization.

Automatic cleaning by means of washer-disinfectors was only carried out at the HPD and HALD in Dakar, Senegal. In France, according to the B.P.P.H., the use of a qualified washer-disinfector is mandatory[27] . Parametric release should be performed by the pharmacist in charge of the sterilization unit. Of the seven hospitals surveyed, only one HPD pharmacist was performing the load validation. The study by DIOUF. W.C, showed the same rate[18] .

In addition to the consequences inherent in the design of practices such as manual washing and the absence of equipment such as washer-disinfectors (washing machines) as well as protective equipment adapted for cleaning (long machete gloves, single-use apron, protective glasses with side shields, etc.) exposes staff to infectious risks....) exposes the staff to infectious risks, this situation was found in most of the sterilization units raising the importance of equipping the sterilization units with washer-disinfectors (washing machine) to avoid outdated and risky practices such as manual washing.

Staff will also need to be provided with protective materials and encouraged to use them. Advocacy for the use of such machines has been done by MILES RS in the UK since 1991[31] . An American study conducted in 2011 that examined new technologies for sterilization and high-level disinfection of critical and semi-critical MDs recommends the use of washer-disinfectors[32] .

V.3.3. The conditioning

Packaging allows the sterile state of the material to be maintained until use. We found that only two hospitals in Senegal practiced secondary packaging of medical devices and surgical textiles. The study by DIOUF. W.C. found the same rate.[18] .

The lack of packaging on M.D. and surgical textiles can lead to recontamination of the sterilized material between the sterilization site and the place of use. Especially since in these hospitals the environment is not protected, this can be a source of contamination (air purification). **Sterilization**

Steam sterilization (autoclave):

The main hospital in Dakar was the only hospital to systematically perform the Bowie Dick test before using the steam sterilizers each morning.

The sterilization tray is the phase during which the chosen temperature is maintained for a specific period of time: for the instrument cycle (metal D.M.) "prions" 134° for 18 minutes; for the elastomer cycle (plastic D.M.) 125° for 20 minutes; for the textile cycle 134° for 10 minutes.

Our results show that only the Hôpital Principal de Dakar respected the temperature and duration of sterilization according to the different types of M.D. and surgical textiles. Some hospitals respected the temperature but not the duration: in Mali, the Point G University Hospital and the Kati University Hospital sterilized their metal M.D.s respectively at a temperature of 134° for 8 minutes and 134° for 5 minutes. In the other hospitals, the temperature and duration were not indicated.

Apart from HPD and CHU-HALD, which sterilized their plastic D.M. by autoclave, the chemical method was used by the other hospitals. The latter proceeded with soaking in the pre-disinfection solution. The dilution of the pre-disinfection solutions recommended by the manufacturers are not often respected at the time of preparation.

It often happens that some hospitals (ENT Department of the CHU-Gabriel Touré Mali) sterilize their metallic DM by soaking, this process is formally banned. However, the study conducted by **Molinari JA et al. In the USA,** over sixteen years of experience with a follow-up of sterilization between 1978 and 1993, showed that 20% of plastic MDs are sterilized by soaking with a chemical solution[22] .

The Bowie Dick test should be performed every morning when the sterilizer is started up before use. This test allows to validate the good penetration of steam in a porous load, i.e. to show the performance of the steam sterilizer.

Daily monitoring of the sterilizer allows the practitioner to be immediately alerted to any malfunctioning and at the same time reduces the risk of infecting a patient with incorrectly sterilized material.

Use of the sterilizer after a non-compliant Bowie Dick test represents a major risk of non-sterility for the loads. Steam sterilization is an effective but delicate and temperamental process that requires maintenance of chamber integrity, good quality generator feed water and careful monitoring of its operation. The sterility of a load is only guaranteed by checking the performance of the sterilizer every morning with a Bowie Dick test.[29] .

Dry heat sterilizer (poupinel):

In Mali, the CHU du Point G and in Senegal the HPD are the only hospitals that do not use the Poupinel for the sterilization of their metallic DM at their central sterilization unit. The study carried out between 1978 and 1993 by **Molinari JA** et al. in France, showed that the Poupinel was used in 10% of cases.[22] . The Poupinel or dry heat sterilizer is today completely ineffective because it is particularly inactive on prions. In France, the Ministry of Health formally advises against its use, if not prohibiting it. Steam sterilization in an autoclave is now the recognized standard in hospitals[22] .

We noted the persistence of the use of dry heat in most of the sterilization units evaluated, which does not guarantee the quality of the sterilization. According to the standards, autoclave sterilization in hospitals is the only recommended process. However, we have observed that the time and pressure of sterilization are not respected, which also compromises the quality of sterilization. To ensure effective sterilization at the sites evaluated, it would be necessary not only to replace all the sterilizers with autoclaves that meet EN NF 285 standards, but also to draw up and apply standard operating procedures (SOPs)

Traceability

Our study has shown that only one hospital has set up a tracking card for the material to be sterilized and this same hospital has carried out the traceability on the M.D. and surgical textiles by providing the following information on the labels (date of sterilization, name of the operator, expiration date, sterilization cycle, identification of the material to be sterilized) the other hospitals have given information on the identification of the material to be sterilized only. However, the study by **SMITH. A.J.** et **All.**, showed that 86% of the surgeries did not have a procedure for the identification and traceability of instruments used on patients[20] .

The installation of steam sterilizers has been qualified in all the selected hospitals in our study, of which only one hospital (14.3%) has written instructions for the operation of these devices. The study by **SMITH. A.J.** et **All.** showed that written instructions for the operation of the sterilizer are not available in 61% of the cases[20] .

Requalification of autoclaves within the required 18-month period

Only one hospital requalified its autoclaves within the required 18-month period (HPD). This same value was found in the study by DIOUF. W.C[18] .

V.4. Quality assurance system

The quality assurance system required by the BPPH, described in Circular No. 672 of October 20, 1997, explains that :

Why? To define the purpose and scope of the procedure.

For whom? List the people involved who are authorized

When? Circumstance of implementation of the procedure

How: Operating procedure, tools to be used, decision criteria

What record? Recording = proof of the application of the procedure

In contrast, the study by **SMITH. A.J. et All.,** found that insurance coverage for sterilizers was available in 79% of cases[20] .

The most recurrent problems in all the sites evaluated concerned the practice of sterilization according to standards.

In addition to defects due to equipment and materials, there are problems related to the quality approach which are transversal, i.e. they concern all stages of sterilization. These include traceability and quality assurance, the implementation of which is imperative for quality sterilization. The sterilization process is not controlled when there is no quality assurance system in the hospital. This results in the release of loads (DM and surgical textiles) which can be a source of nosocomial infection.

V.5. The personnel of the sterilization units.

The majority of the sterilization units were run by physicians, whereas the standards recommend that they be run by pharmacists.

Among the staff, laborers and orderlies were more involved in sterilization process activities than other health care managers, although the standards that specify staff qualification for these activities do not mention this occupational category (Table X).

Only the main hospital in Dakar had subjected these agents to continuous training. We found that compared to European data, both countries need to make an effort to improve the quality of the sterilization process. For example, **SHAH et al.** in 2007 found that 88% of European ministries supported staff training on sterilization.

That of **SMITH. A.J et al.** was similar to our result.[20] .

We found that no pharmacist was designated to manage the sterilization units.

In Senegal, two of the three hospitals surveyed are managed by pharmacists.

For better coordination of sterilization activities, management should be entrusted to the in-house pharmacy by appointing a pharmacist as unit manager.

Of the seven hospitals, only HPD has trained these agents in good sterilization practices. In addition, it organizes ongoing training for these agents once a week through theoretical courses and practical cases encountered during the week. On the other hand, the study by **SHAH. R et al,** showed that 88% of the departments provided training in cross-infection control to their sterilization department staff[19] , the study by **SMITH. A.J** et **al,** was similar to our result.[20] .

Two hospitals in Senegal (HPD and HALD) organized medical visits for their sterilization unit agents. However, the study by DIOUF W.C. obtained a rate of 57.1%. [18].

The staff of the sterilization unit, although exposed, have never received appropriate vaccination as part of their activities in Mali and Senegal. However, the study by **SHAH. R** et **al.** reported that 98% of ministries have a policy to check the vaccination status of staff[19] .

The fight against nosocomial infections is a constant battle. The constant appearance of new sources of contamination and the lack of knowledge of some of them, requires a permanent questioning of the means of control used and their evolution. The treatment of reusable medical devices, and sterilization in particular, represent an essential element in the fight against nosocomial infections, which are a problem and a threat to public health.

Sterilization failure is possible at all levels from the architectural design of the sterilization unit, the steps of the sterilization process to the quality assurance system.

This work has allowed us to evaluate the respect of the BPS in the different health structures, not only to have an idea on the practice of the principle of the forward march and also of the process of the sterilization of the M.D. and operating textiles. To do this, we conducted a survey that focused on the essential points of the sterilization of M.D. and surgical textiles that could allow us to appreciate the practices of sterilization and their relative behavior compared to the standards required in this area. This study was therefore conducted to highlight these shortcomings in selected hospitals in Mali and Senegal in order to propose corrective measures. These hospitals were selected in a representative way and evaluated by an observation method and an analysis of the gaps with the recommended standards, which made it possible to identify the following major problems

- The architectural design does not allow for the forward motion circuit.
- The steps of the sterilization process were not respected on the majority of our sterilization units.
- The quality assurance system was not implemented at any of the facilities in our study.
- Lack of PSR training for agents involved in the sterilization process

At the end of this work, the important points regarding sterilization represented by the results of our study showed that in Mali, no sterilization unit was attached to the internal use pharmacy in accordance with the standards in force. However, in Senegal, only one (1/3) sterilization unit was attached to the internal use pharmacy (HPD).

The architecture of the premises of the central sterilization units must allow, whenever possible, the respect of the principle of forward movement.

In our study, the Hôpital Principal de Dakar was the only hospital to have a washer-disinfector with a technical wall that allowed the forward circuit to be respected.

The surface area of the sterilization units was insufficient in all the hospitals included in our study in Mali. Our findings revealed that in Senegal the surface area of the sterilization unit was sufficient in only one hospital. However, it should be noted that the sterilization unit was easy to clean in only one hospital in Senegal (HPD).

The distribution circuit did not make it possible to avoid re-contamination of the M.D. and surgical textiles in any of the sterilization units in Mali. However, in Senegal, the distribution circuit was respected in only 1/3 of the hospitals (HPD).

Immediate soaking after use of the MDs was performed in 3/7 hospitals in both countries (2/4 hospitals in Mali and 1/3 in Senegal). Immediate soaking avoids blood clotting on the MDs in order to prevent the formation of bio-film. We found that the other 4/7 (57.1%) sterilization units received the MDs wrapped in surgical drapes for transport from the OR to the sterilization unit.

Products that comply with current standards for the pre-disinfection of MDs were available in 2/4 hospitals in Mali and 1/3 hospital in Senegal.

According to the **NF EN ISO 15 883-2** standard, manual washing is no longer recommended, although our survey showed that the majority of sterilization units carry out manual washing using brushes. In addition, we observed that outside of the Hôpital Principal de Dakar, staff do not use the protective equipment recommended for this operation, such as long-sleeved gloves, protective aprons, goggles, masks, and clogs. In Senegal, only two hospitals practiced secondary packaging of medical devices and surgical textiles, of which one hospital had all the necessary protective equipment for its staff.

The main hospital in Dakar was the only hospital to systematically perform the Bowie Dick test before using the steam sterilizers each morning.

Sterilization of metallic D.M. :

Metal MDs were sterilized with the steam sterilizer in 2/4 hospitals in Mali. But in Senegal, all hospitals sterilized their metallic MDs with the steam sterilizer.

In Mali, the 134° for 18 minutes cycle was not used for sterilization of metallic DM. CHU-Kati used the 134° for 8 minutes cycle, CHU-Point used 134° for 5 minutes. It should be noted that in Senegal, the 134° for 18 minutes cycle was used in only 1/3 of the hospitals. We have no information on the sterilization cycle of the other 2/3 sterilization units.

Textile sterilization: We found that only two sterilization units sterilized their surgical textiles in accordance with the time and pressure standards in force in both countries (CHU-Gabriel Touré in Mali with a cycle of 134° for 13 minutes and HPD in Senegal with a cycle of 134° for 10 minutes).

Sterilization of plastic MDs: In Mali, none of the hospitals in our study sterilized their plastic MDs with steam. In Senegal, only 1/3 of the hospitals sterilized their plastic MDs at a cycle of 125° for a period of 20 minutes according to the standards.

Among the hospitals surveyed, we found that only 1/7 (14.3%) hospitals do not have a sterilization unit. It does not sterilize their metal DM with dry heat.

All the 7/7 sterilization units have proceeded to the qualification of their sterilization equipment at their facilities. Only one of these sterilization units has proceeded with the requalification of its autoclaves within the required 18 months 1/7.

The quality assurance system required by the BPPH according to circular N° 672 of October 20, 1997 did not exist in any of the sterilization departments of the hospitals included in our study.

The head of the sterilization unit was a pharmacist in a single hospital in Senegal.

Laborers were involved in sterilization activities in three-quarters of the hospitals, i.e., 25.0% of the staff categories in Mali. The staff dedicated to the sterilization unit did not receive any basic training, periodic medical check-ups of the staff were never performed, and no appropriate vaccinations were carried out in the context of their activities.

In Senegal, laborers were involved in sterilization activities in only one sterilization unit, and apart from the HPD sterilization unit staff, the staff in the other sterilization units did not receive any basic training in compliance with GHP, and 2/3 of the hospitals organized medical visits once a year for the sterilization unit staff (HALD and HPD). As in Mali, none of the sterilization unit staff received appropriate vaccination as part of their activities. We can see that among the different stages of the sterilization process, efforts still need to be made. Overall, even if the authorities are aware of the importance of good sterilization, there are still gaps to be filled, as we have just seen, and this is what has allowed us to make some recommendations in this regard:

Hospitals in Mali and Senegal will need to be upgraded, which will certainly require significant investment, but it must be admitted that "the sterility of a product is not negotiable, as the safety of the patient is not negotiable. This will include training of sterilization service agents, installation of adequate equipment (autoclaves, washer-disinfectors, etc.) that meets current international standards, and construction or rehabilitation of units in accordance with architectural requirements. It is also necessary to develop a regulatory and legislative arsenal to govern the practice of sterilization, with texts adapted to the local context and in phase with the policy of these two countries.

In the future, it could be envisaged to use exclusively single-use material. However, this solution does not seem economically relevant. Another possible approach would be to outsource the sterilization and disinfection of equipment. It would therefore be useful to measure the financial and organizational impact of such a choice for a hospital structure.

The main recommendations are shown in the following table (Table XXI):

Table XXI: RECOMMENDATION

OBSERVATIONS	RECOMMENDATION	COUNTRIES AND HOSPITALS CONCERNED	DG	R.U.S	P.U.S
No central sterilization unit has been attached to the in-house pharmacy.	Attach the central sterilization units to the internal use pharmacy and give management to a pharmacist.	**Mali :** CHU-Gabriel Touré, Point-G, Kati and Hôpital Luxemboug **Senegal**: HOGGY Hospital, A Le Dantec	X		
Some pharmacists have not received specific training on sterilization, i.e. Good Sterilization Practices	Train all pharmacists in the internal use pharmacy on good sterilization practices.	**Mali :** CHU-Gabriel Touré, Point-G, Kati and Hôpital Luxemboug **Senegal:** Aristide Le Dantec Hospital, HOGGY, Principal of Dakar	X	X	
Only one pharmacist was head of the sterilization unit	Give responsibility for the sterilization unit to the pharmacist	**Mali :** CHU-Gabriel Touré, Point-G, Kati and Hôpital Luxemboug **Senegal:** Aristide Le Dantec Hospital, HOGGY	X		
some sterilization unit staff have not received appropriate initial training in BPS	Train the sterilization unit staff on BPS.	CHU-Gabriel Touré, Point-G, Kati and Hôpital Luxemboug **Senegal:** Aristide Le Dantec Hospital, HOGGY,	X	X	
Some sterilization unit workers have never received periodic medical check-ups and appropriate vaccinations as part of their activities	Organize periodic medical visits to the sterilization unit agents and have them vaccinated	**Mali :** CHU-Gabriel Touré, Point-G, Kati and Hôpital Luxemboug **Senegal:** Aristide Le Dantec Hospital, HOGGY, Principal of Dakar	X	X	X
In addition to the activities of the sterilization unit, staff also work in the operating room to assist the surgeons and perform routine nursing shifts at the hospital	Detach staff from the sterilization unit to the sterilization department only in order to carry out their activities, thus minimizing the risk of re-contamination.	**Mali :** CHU-Gabriel Touré, Point-G, Kati and Hôpital Luxemboug **Senegal:** Aristide Le Dantec Hospital, HOGGY,	X		
The means of protection for the personnel of a sterilization unit should not be the ordinary gloves only	Make available, in addition to ordinary gloves, household gloves, goggles, single-use aprons, clogs, masks for the protection of personnel	**Mali :** CHU-Gabriel Touré, Point-G, Kati and Hôpital Luxemboug **Senegal:** Aristide Le Dantec Hospital, HOGGY,	X	X	

Table XXI: RECOMMENDATION (continued1)

Point to improve	recommendation		DG	R.U.S	P.U.S
some washing areas were not equipped with cabins and washing machines	in addition to the sinks, equip the washing areas with washing cabins and provide at least one washing machine for DM	**Mali :** CHU-Gabriel Touré, Point-G, Kati and Hôpital Luxemboug **Senegal:** HOGGY Hospital	X		
The production areas were not separated by technical walls	Separate the different production areas in order to maintain the sterile state of the sterilized DM and surgical textiles in compliance with the BPS	**Mali :** CHU-Gabriel Touré, Point-G, Kati and Hôpital Luxemboug **Senegal:** Aristide Le Dantec Hospital, HOGGY	X		
The forward march was not respected according to the BPS	Respect the forward circuit in order to maintain the sterile state of the M.D.	**Mali :** CHU-Gabriel Touré, Point-G, Kati and Hôpital Luxemboug **Senegal:** Aristide Le Dantec Hospital, HOGGY, Principal of Dakar	X	X	X
Secondary packaging did not exist in some hospitals and even if it did, it was not often used on DM and surgical drapes.	Make secondary packaging available and practice secondary packaging on DM and textiles in order to maintain the sterile state until distribution.	**Mali :** CHU-Gabriel Touré, Point-G, Kati and Hôpital Luxemboug **Senegal:** Aristide Le Dantec Hospital, HOGGY	X	X	X
the packaging areas contain materials that can be a source of contamination.	Do not place materials that may be a source of contamination in production areas	**Mali :** CHU-Gabriel Touré, Point-G, Kati and Hôpital Luxemboug **Senegal:** Aristide Le Dantec Hospital, HOGGY		X	X
Some hospitals did not have tape with a pass-through indicator, as well as heat sealers for sealing DM.	Make available the tape with a passage indicator and heat sealer for the sealing of DM	**Mali :** CHU-Gabriel Touré, Point-G	X	X	
The reception of soiled DM and the distribution of sterilized DM were not separated.	Separate the circuit of reception of soiled DM and distribution of sterilized DM in order to avoid recontamination and to maintain the sterile state.	**Mali :** CHU-Gabriel Touré, Point-G, Kati and Hôpital Luxemboug **Senegal:** Aristide Le Dantec Hospital, HOGGY	X		

Table XXI: RECOMMENDATION (continued2)

Point to improve	recommendation		DG	R.U.S	P.U.S
Hospitals have not implemented a protocol for the pre-disinfection of DM in accordance with the standards	Make the DM pre-disinfection protocol available to sterilization unit agents and posted wherever needed.	**Mali :** CHU-Gabriel Touré, Pcint-G, Kati and Hôpital Luxemboug **Senegal:** Aristide Le Dantec Hospital, HOGGY	X	X	
Some hospitals do not have products that comply with the current standards or even if these products exist they mix it with bleach,	Use products that comply with current standards and never mix with bleach,	**Mali :** CHU-Gabriel Touré, Pcint-G, Kati and Hôpital Luxemboug **Senegal:** Aristide Le Dantec Hospital, HOGGY	X	X	X
The dilution and soaking time of the DM and pre-disinfection products were not respected.	Respect the dilution and soaking time of the products used for the pre-disinfection of MD.	**Mali :** CHU-Gabriel Touré, Pcint-G, Kati and Hôpital Luxemboug **Senegal:** Aristide Le Dantec Hospital, HOGGY		X	X
Some hospitals did not soak the MDs in the pre-disinfection solution right after the operation in the operating room	Immediately soak the soiled DMs in the OR in closed bins right after interventions before sending them to the US	**Mali :** CHU-Gabriel Touré, Pcint-G, Kati and Hôpital Luxemboug **Senegal:** Aristide Le Dantec Hospital, HOGGY		X	
The Bowie Dick test was not performed before using the autoclave	Use the Bowie Dick test every day before using the autoclave	**Mali :** CHU-Gabriel Touré, Point-G, Kati and Hôpital Luxemboug **Senegal:** Aristide Le Dantec Hospital, HOGGY		X	X
Some sterilization units do not have steam sterilizers that comply with EN NF 285 standards	Provide steam sterilizers that comply with EN NF 285 standards	**Mali :** CHU-Gabriel Touré, and Hôpital Luxemboug **Senegal:** Aristide Le Dantec Hospital, HOGGY	X		
Some hospitals did not sterilize their metal and plastic DMs in the autoclave (or the cycles were not respected)	Sterilize metallic and plastic DM in autoclave respecting the cycle of 134° during 18min for metallic DM and 125° during 10min for plastic DM	**Mali :** CHU-Gabriel Touré, Point-G, Kati and Hôpital Luxemboug **Senegal:** Aristide Le Dantec Hospital, HOGGY		X	X

Table XXI: RECOMMENDATION (continued)

Point to improve	recommendation		DG	R.U.S	P.U.S
The poupinel has been used in most hospitals for the sterilization of metallic DM.	Stop the use of sterilization poupinels for the sterilization of metallic DM or respect the cycle of 180° during 60 minutes	**Mali :** CHU-Gabriel Touré, Point-G, Kati and Hôpital Luxemboug **Senegal:** Aristide Le Dantec Hospital, HOGGY	X	X	X
Some sterilizers have not been requalified within the required timeframe (every 18 months)	Re-qualification of autoclaves within the 18-month timeframe	**Mali :** CHU-Gabriel Touré, Point-G, Kati and Hôpital Luxemboug **Senegal:** Aristide Le Dantec Hospital, HOGGY	X		
The quality assurance system has not been implemented in hospitals for sterilization units	Implement the quality assurance system in the sterilization department one	**Mali :** CHU-Gabriel Touré, Point-G, Kati and Hôpital Luxemboug **Senegal:** Aristide Le Dantec Hospital, HOGGY, Principal of Dakar	X		
The labeling did not include all relevant information	Put all the necessary information on the D.M. and operating textiles at the time of labelling.	**Mali :** CHU-Gabriel Touré, Point-G, Kati and Hôpital Luxemboug **Senegal:** Aristide Le Dantec Hospital, HOGGY		X	X
Management supports for traceability and non-compliance were not available.	Provide staff with management tools for traceability and non-compliance	**Mali :** CHU-Gabriel Touré, Point-G, Kati and Hôpital Luxemboug **Senegal:** Aristide Le Dantec Hospital, HOGGY		X	X
The tracking sheets were non-existent for the materials to be sterilized	Set up tracking sheets for materials to be sterilized	**Mali :** CHU-Gabriel Touré, Point-G, Kati and Hôpital Luxemboug **Senegal:** Aristide Le Dantec Hospital, HOGGY		X	

OUTLOOK

Set up a good sterilization circuit while respecting the BPS and BPPH.

In our study, it was not possible to take samples from the sterilized equipment for analysis of the microorganisms responsible for nosocomial infections (bactericides, virucides and fungicides). In order to assess the effectiveness of pre-disinfection and the entire sterilization process on the DM and surgical textiles in the hospital. A study carried out in this sense could contribute effectively to the fight against nosocomial infections.

REFERENCES

1. DUBAELE MP

Hospital sterilization certified by an organization. Phar thesis, University of Paris-Sud, Faculty of Pharmacy of Chatenay-Malabry, France 2000. P.5

2. RIHOUEY. G.B

Sterilization, Quality Manager - Pharmacy Unit. CHU. ROUEN, France, 2007, P2-3-4-7

3. KHBIZA. S.Y

Organization of a centralized sterilization unit at the Sidi Lahcen hospital in the prefecture of SKHIRAT-TEMARA, dissertation MS Morocco, 2004-2006, P.1

4. GOULLET. D

The notion of "sterile", Nice, 16 and 17 April 1997. Text updated on January 13, 2006. Revue de L'ADPHSO - Tome 22 n°3, Lyon, France, 1997 - pp37-45.

5. VALENCIA. B

Steam sterilization (Autoclave), CCLIN magazine, Grenoble, France ? 2010. P.3

6. NF EN 556-2 (AFS) STANDARD

Sterilization of medical devices - Requirements for medical devices to be labelled "sterile" - Part 2: Requirements for aseptically prepared medical devices (Classification number: S 98-107-2), July 2004, http://afs.asso.fr/cms/index.php

7. NF EN 285 STANDARD (AFNOR)

Related to sterilization. Steam sterilizers: large sterilizers.
CEFH, February 1997

8. TARI C, RISSE A, MOLL P, RIERA Y, ROLLET D

The role of sterilization in the fight against nosocomial infections, IBODE, Toulin, version 12 06 2009. P1

9. NF EN 1040

Antiseptics and chemical disinfectants - Basic bactericidal activity of antiseptics - Test method and prescription (phase 1), April 2006 AFNOR éditeur, Paris pp. 1-43.

10. NATIONAL AGENCY FOR THE SAFETY OF MEDICINES AND HEALTH PRODUCTS

Definition of Medical Device (MD), http://www. ansm. sante.fr/Produits-de- sante/Dispositifs-medicaux accessed June 03, 2012

11. LAROUSSE FRENCH DICTIONARY

Sterilizer definition,

www.larousse.fr/dictionnaires/francais/stérilisateur/74669, **accessed June 03, 2012**

12. BERGHEAU F, GOULLET D

French and European Regulations and Recommendations on Sterilization, AFS editor, Paris, 27 01 2011.

13. HUYS J

Sterilization   cycle,   WFHSS   forum,   updated   on   26   March   2012 http://www.wfhss.com/html/educ/sbasics/sbasics01 en.htm accessed on 03 06 2012

14. NF EN 13727

Antiseptic and chemical disinfectants - Quantitative suspension test for the evaluation of the bactericidal activity of chemical disinfectants for instruments used in medicine - Test method and requirements (phase 2, step 1) (bactericidia under soiled conditions) Lyon, July 2004

15. NF EN 13624

Antiseptic and chemical disinfectants - Quantitative suspension test for the evaluation of the fungicidal activity of chemical disinfectants used for instruments in medicine - Test method and requirements (phase 2, step 1) yeasticidal activity, limited to Candida albicans) Lyon, April 2004

16. DIU of Hospital Sterilization

DIU01 pre-disinfection and cleaning " Acquisition of knowledge " definition pre-disinfection, Reception and sorting, Packaging, sterilization Lyon and Grenoble, updated on 06 / 09 / 2010.

17. DIU of Hospital Sterilization

DIU06 Quality approach " Acquisition of knowledge " definition Process Lyon and Grenoble.

18. DIOUF W.C

Survey on the practices of sterilization of DM in hospitals in the Dakar Region, Pharm thesis, December 2009.

19. SHAH R, COLLINS. JM, HODE. TM, LAING. ER.

A national study of cross infection control: are we clean enough? *Br Dent J.* 2007; 203(8):E16.

20. SMITH AJ, BAGG J, HURRELL D, MCHUGH S.

Sterilization of re-usable instruments in general dental practice. Br Dent J. 2007;203(8):E16

21. BAGG. J, SMITH. A.J, HURRELL. D, McHUGH. S, IRVINE. G.

Pre-sterilization cleaning of re-usable instruments in general dental practice, British Dental Journal (*Br Dent J). 2007;202(9) :550-1,,*

22. MOLINARI JA, GLEASON MJ, MERCHANT VA

Sixteen years of experience with sterilization monitoring. Compendium. 1994 Dec;15(12):1422-4, 1426-8 passim; quiz 1432.

23. AUPEE M., GOETZ M.L

Sterilization and hospital hygiene " Sterilization in hospitals ". Published by the European Center for Health Services. CEFH, 1998, Paris, pp. 58-59.

24. GOULLET D,

Interest and Good Practices of the decontamination of the medical-surgical material.

Le pharmacien hospitalier, 1992, 27, N° 110, pp. 13-22.

25. GIP FCIP - CAFOC of the Academy of Toulouse

sterilization agent in a hospital environment" Official Journal 2011, NSF Code 331s

26. DARBORD JC, Désinfection et stérilisation dans les établissements de soins, 5ème edition, Masson, Paris, 2003, pp. 85

27. CHAUMEIL JC, ANTIGNAC S, AULAGNER G, BERNHEIM C, BRANDON M, CALLANQUIN M et al.

Good Hospital Pharmacy Practices, 1ère edition, France 2001. P.42

28. MEUNIER J

Good sterilization practices, steam sterilizers for permeable loads, Central Market Commission, G.P.E.M./S.L., Edition (2000), France, P.62

29. Hygiene and Sterilization Recommendation Guides by the Department of Health

http://www.medical-hygiene.com/Files/28696/mediawebserver.pdf, accessed July 9, 2012.

30. RS MILES

What standards should we use for the disinfection of large equipment? J Hosp Infect. 1991 Jun; 18 Suppl A:264-73

31. RUTALA WA, WEBER DJ

Sterilization, high-level disinfection, and environmental cleaning, Infect Dis Clin North Am. 2011 Mar;25(1):45-76.

Summary

To contribute to the fight against nosocomial infections in the context of better patient care in hospitals, a study was conducted to evaluate the sterilization processes for reusable medical devices and surgical drapes in seven hospitals in Mali and Senegal.

This study was conducted in the sterilization units of four hospitals in Mali and three in Senegal. It was a descriptive study of the process of sterilization of reusable DM and surgical drapes in these hospital structures. The work took place between September 15 and November 15, 2011 for the surveys conducted in Mali and from December 1, 2011 to January 31, 2012 for those conducted in Senegal.
A total of 7 sterilization departments were evaluated in the 7 hospitals in both countries
These assessments found that in both countries only one CSSD was attached to the hospital pharmacy and that 28.6% of the heads of the sterilization departments or units were pharmacists. These results revealed that 85.7% of the staff had never received basic BPS training. The surface area of the sterilization departments or units was insufficient in 85.7% of the cases, leading to the observation that the "forward" principle was respected in only 14.3% of the departments evaluated. Cleaning and disinfection products conforming to standards were available in 42.9% of hospitals. Secondary packaging was used in 28.6% of the sterilization units. In Mali, 50% of the hospitals sterilized their metal sterile goods with steam, whereas in Senegal we found that all hospitals sterilized their metal sterile goods with steam. No sterilization service evaluated in either country had yet implemented a quality assurance system for the activities conducted.
The shortcomings identified made it possible to formulate recommendations for better treatment of DM and surgical fields, which will make it possible to strengthen the sterilization services and units in Mali and Senegal. This will contribute to the improvement of the quality of care.

Key words : Sterilization, DM, operating textiles, Hospital, Sterilization unit

APPENDICES
ANNEX N°1 QUESTIONNAIRE

Country: ....
City: ....
Hospital: ....
Service: ....

I. Identification of the sterilization service:
To which department is the sterilization unit attached?
At Hospital Pharmacy □
In the Operating   Room□
At   Surgery□
Other to be   specified□
II. Identification of personnel (human resources)
    a. Is the department head of the sterilization unit:
A   Physician□
A   Pharmacist□
A senior health technician □
A Medical Assistant   □
Other to be specified   □
    b. Do the sterilization agents include :
Pharmacist(s)   □
Physician(s)   □
Senior health technician(s) □
Medical Assistant(s)   □
Volunteer(s)   □
Pharmacy Preparers   □
Maneuver(s)   □
Other to be specified□Are these staff dedicated to sterilization only: yes□no   □
Is a supervisory cadre (Major) appointed for sterilization: yes □ no □ Have agents
received initial training in sterilization: yes□no□
    c. Do dedicated sterilization staff receive periodic medical checkups: yes □ no □
    d. Are you vaccinated to do this job? : yes □ no □
Does the staff have the means of protection against the risks of contamination related to
the treatment of DM and surgical fields such as: Ordinary gloves   □
Household gloves   □
Single-use apron □
Safety glasses □
Clog   □
III. Identification of the sterilization unit
Does the central sterilization unit in the hospital have..:
A dirty area □
A clean area □
A sterile area[1] -[1]
A locker room   □
A relaxation room □

A storage area for sterilized materials □
Other area to be specified □
Architectural design:
Is sterilization centralized at your hospital: yes □ no □
Position of the central sterilization unit in the OR
Building housing the block □
Close to the   block□
Away from the block   □
Does the size of the sterilization unit seem to you? :
Sufficient □
Insufficient □

Are the surfaces smooth
Yes   □
No   □
Are the surfaces easy to clean
Yes   □
                    No□
Is the forward march respected: yes □ no □
Is the wash area equipped with :
Drainer   ,□
Sink   ,□
Sink,   □
Washing machine, □
Packaging area:
Are the different production areas (dirty area and clean area) separated by a technical
wall: yes   □□
Are the different production areas (clean area and sterile area) separated by a technical
wall: yes □ no □
Does the packaging area contain materials that could be a source of contamination? : yes
□ no □
Do you have tape with a passing indicator: yes □ no □
Do you have a heat sealer: yes □ no □
Storage area
Does the storage area contain metal shelving: or □ no □
Equipment or material available for sterilization
Autoclave :
Number of autoclaves available ________//
Poupinel:
Number of dolls available ___________//
IV. Identification of the medical devices and reusable surgical fields circuit:
Is the receipt of soiled instruments and the distribution of sterilized instruments separate? :
yes □ no □
Do distribution conditions for sterilized DMs prevent recontamination? : yes □ no □
V. Pre-disinfection. Cleaning
Pre-disinfection
Is there a pre-disinfection protocol for DM and surgical drapes: yes □ no □
What type of product is used for the pre-disinfection of DM :

Products that comply with current standards □
Other products used to   specify□
Is DM soaking performed immediately after surgery: yes □ no □
If not, under what conditions are the DMs sent for sterilization?
In bins with lids   □
Transport Cabinets   □
Other to be specified for the transport of
Does the decontamination bin conform to the volume of the equipment: yes □ no □
Is the decontamination bin graduated: yes □ no □
Is the dilution during pre-disinfection correct: yes □ no □
Are articulated instruments opened and or disassembled before soaking: yes o no □
After pre-disinfection is the equipment rinsed: yes □ no □
Cleaning
What washing process do you use? :
Washing with the washing machine □
Washing cabin with water pressure for carts and containers □
Manual washing □
If yes, what type of equipment is used for cleaning :
Brush □
Sponge □

VI. Identification of sterilization methods

Do you practice secondary packaging: yes □ no □
Is the Bowie Dick test performed before using the autoclave: **yes** □ no □ If yes what cycle do you use? : 134° for 3.5 minutes
Other cycles to be specified ....
Does the sterilization unit have steam sterilizers that comply with EN NF 285 yes □ no □
If so have they qualified: yes □ no □
Are metal DMs sterilized with steam? : yes □ no □ If yes what sterilization cycle do you use: 134° for 18 minutes: yes □ no □ Other cycles please specify:
Are DMs sterilized with dry heat? : yes □ no □ If yes what sterilization cycle do you use: 180° for 60 minutes: yes □ no □ Other cycles please specify:
Are surgical textiles steam sterilized? : yes □ no □
If yes to which sterilization cycle do you use: 134° for 10 minutes: yes □ no □ Other cycles please specify: ....
Are plastic DMs sterilized with steam? : yes □ no □ If yes what sterilization cycle do you use: 125° for 20 minutes: yes □ no □ Other temperature to specify:
Does the sterilization unit process material from another facility: yes □ no □
Are sterilizers requalified within the required time frame (every 18 months): yes no   □□
Are sterilized loads subject to parametric release: yes □ no □
If so, which parameters are monitored?
Verification that packages are free of moisture: yes □ no □ Verification of pass-through indicators: yes □ no □ Verification of package integrity: yes □ no □ Is distribution of sterile material performed immediately after sterilization: yes □ no □
If not, where are the sterilized medical devices stored?
Does the sterilization department have a quality assurance system: yes □ no □

VII. Labeling:
Are sterilized DMs and surgical drapes labeled: yes □ no □ If yes does the label include the
following information: Date of sterilization: yes □ no □
Expiration date: yes□ no □
   Operator name: yes□ no □
   Equipment identification: yes □ no □
   Is there Integrator Archiving: yes □ no □
VIII. Non-compliance management:
   Is there a record book of noncompliance of sterilized materials: yes □ no □
   Recording of non-compliance are they done in writing: yes □ no □
   Recording of non-compliance is done how:
                 Register□
                 Leaf□
Computer Science [1]
IX.traceability :
   Is there a log available to record the traceability of sterilized materials: yes □ no □
   Is there a tracking sheet for equipment to be sterilized: yes □ no □

HOPITAL DU POINT G
BAMAKO

Document de cycle

Stérilisateur :	SELECTOMAT 2	Nom Opérateur :	
Date :	08/04/2008		
Programme :	UNIVERSEL		
Numéro de cycle :	174	Dernier Test B&D :	n°32 12/12/2007 12:03:23
Durée du cycle :	00:43:52	Dernier Test Vide :	n°24 04/12/2007 10:59:52

Pré-Traitement	Plateau	Séchage

Pré-Traitement

- 11:37:58 Préparation
Fin Phase :   981 mbar
- 11:38:10 Vide
Fin Phase :   65 mbar
- 11:41:14 Balayage de vapeur
Fin Phase :   79 mbar
- 11:42:17 Injection de vapeur
Fin Phase :   1488 mbar
- 11:44:04 Vide
Fin Phase :   79 mbar
- 11:46:32 Balayage de vapeur
Fin Phase :   92 mbar
- 11:47:36 Injection de vapeur
Fin Phase :   1000 mbar
- 11:48:41 Vide
Fin Phase :   78 mbar
- 11:50:33 Balayage de vapeur
Fin Phase :   90 mbar
- 11:51:37 Chauffage
Fin Phase :   3100 mbar

Plateau

Début	Fin	Durée
11:56:56	12:01:59	00:05:03

	Temp.	Pression
Début	135	3100
Fin	135	3089
Mini	135	3085
Maxi	135,3	3112
Moy.	135,2	3098,4

Variation Temp.:   0,3 °C
Variation Press.:   27 mbar
Fo :   163

Séchage

- 12:01:58 Détente de pression
Fin Phase :   148 mbar
- 12:05:03 Séchage
Fin Phase :   63 mbar
- 12:07:05 Aération intermédiaire
Fin Phase :   953 mbar
- 12:08:35 Séchage
Fin Phase :   67 mbar
- 12:12:01 Aération intermédiaire
Fin Phase :   955 mbar
- 12:13:31 Séchage
Fin Phase :   62 mbar
- 12:16:53 Aération intermédiaire
Fin Phase :   955 mbar
- 12:18:23 Séchage
Fin Phase :   111 mbar
- 12:20:05 Aération
Fin Phase :   912 mbar
- 12:20:49 Retrait joint de porte
Fin Phase :   956 mbar
- 12:21:50 Fin de programme
Fin Phase :   956 mbar

Fin de programme

Validé par :

HOPITAL DU POINT G
BAMAKO

Document de cycle

Stérilisateur :	SELECTOMAT 2	Nom Opérateur :	
Date :	07/04/2008		
Programme :	UNIVERSEL		
Numéro de cycle :	172	Dernier Test B&D :	n°32 12/12/2007 12:03:23
Durée du cycle :	00:45:51	Dernier Test Vide :	n°24 04/12/2007 10:59:52

INVALIDE

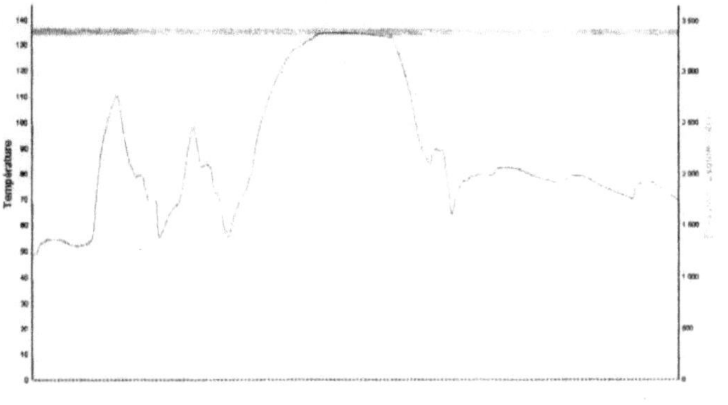

Pré-Traitement	Plateau	Séchage

Pré-Traitement

- 15:13:56 Préparation
Fin Phase :   973 mbar
- 15:14:10 Vide
Fin Phase :   63 mbar
- 15:17:07 Balayage de vapeur
Fin Phase :   61 mbar
- 15:18:11 Injection de vapeur
Fin Phase :   1483 mbar
- 15:19:59 Vide
Fin Phase :   78 mbar
- 15:23:18 Balayage de vapeur
Fin Phase :   90 mbar
- 15:24:22 Injection de vapeur
Fin Phase :   953 mbar
- 15:25:27 Vide
Fin Phase :   78 mbar
- 15:26:02 Balayage de vapeur
Fin Phase :   92 mbar
- 15:29:07 Chauffage
Fin Phase :   3007 mbar

Plateau

Début	Fin	Durée
15:34:26	15:39:26	00:05:00

	Temp.	Pression
Début	134,9	3097
Fin	133,4	3085
Mini	133,4	3084
Maxi	135,2	3108
Moy.	134,8	3095,7

Variation Temp.:	1,8 °C
Variation Press.:	24 mbar
Fo :	151

Séchage

- 15:39:25 Détente de pression
Fin Phase :   149 mbar
- 15:43:01 Séchage
Fin Phase :   63 mbar
- 15:45:04 Aération intermédiaire
Fin Phase :   949 mbar
- 15:46:34 Séchage
Fin Phase :   65 mbar
- 15:49:57 Aération intermédiaire
Fin Phase :   949 mbar
- 15:51:27 Séchage
Fin Phase :   57 mbar
- 15:54:50 Aération intermédiaire
Fin Phase :   953 mbar
- 15:56:20 Séchage
Fin Phase :   103 mbar
- 15:58:03 Aération
Fin Phase :   908 mbar
- 15:58:46 Retrait joint de porte
Fin Phase :   953 mbar
- 15:59:48 Fin de programme
Fin Phase :   953 mbar

Fin de programme

Validé par :

ANNEXE 3

QUELQUES IMAGES DES UNITES DE STERILISATION

Zone sale (zone de lavage) :

Lavage manuel effectué avec brosse, utilisation d'eau de javel et cotol

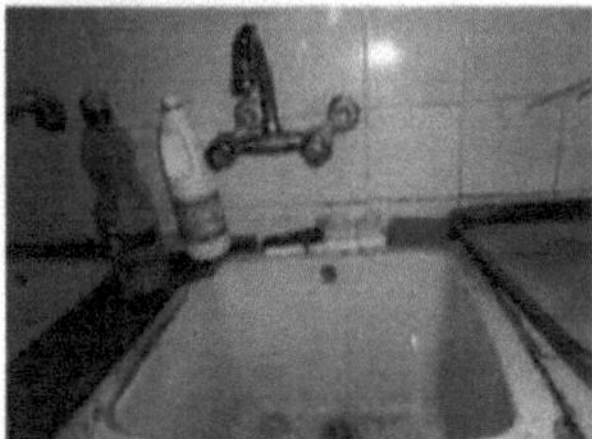

Zone propre (Zone de conditionnement) :

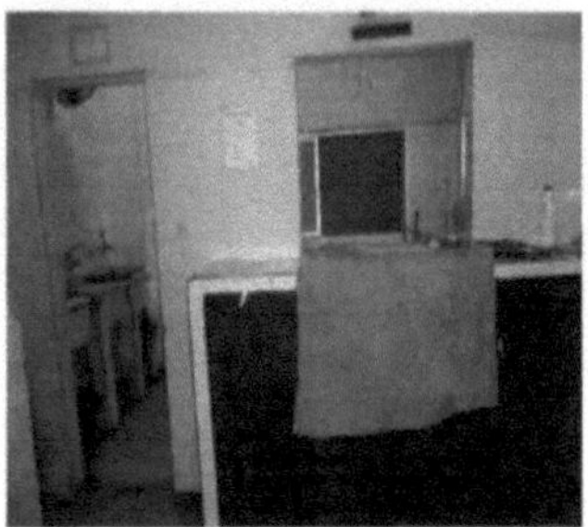

Zone propre (zone de conditionnement)

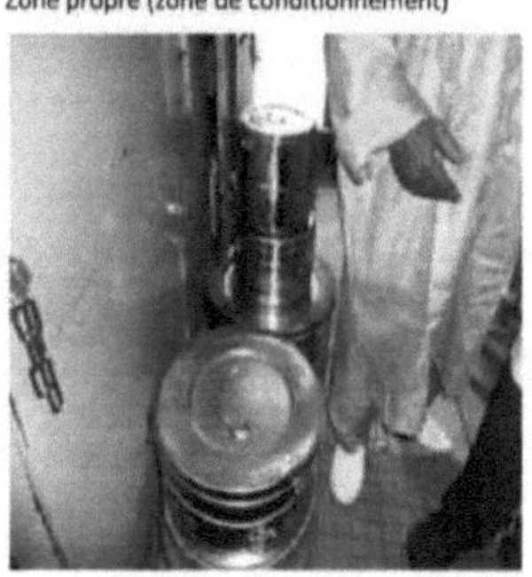

Zone propre (zone de conditionnement)

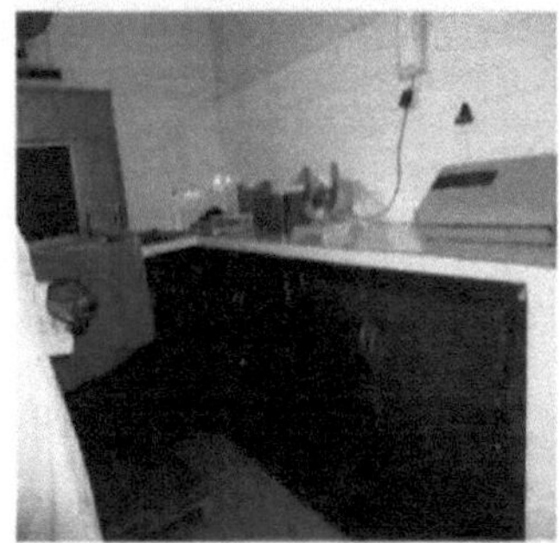

Autoclave

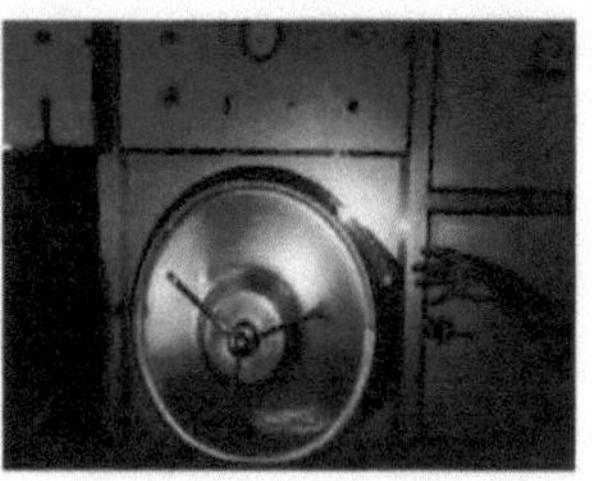

Autoclave

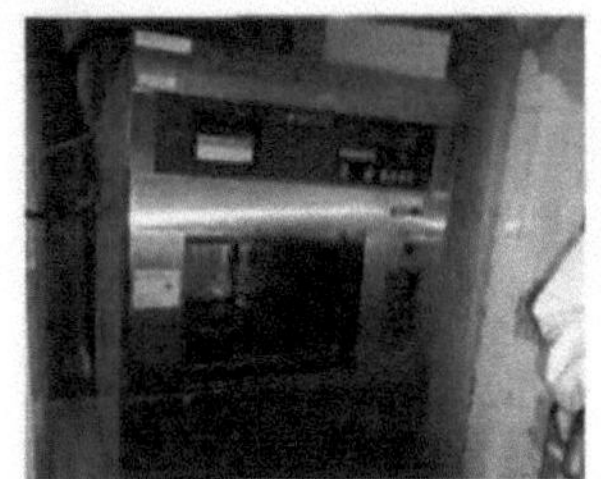

ANNEXE 3

QUELQUES IMAGES DES UNITES DE STERILISATION

Poupinel

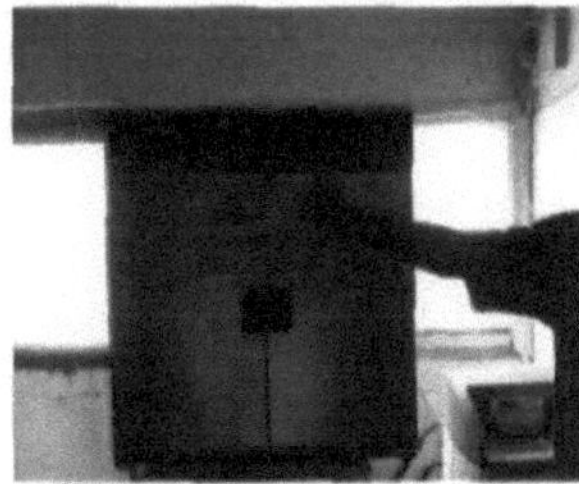

Poupinel

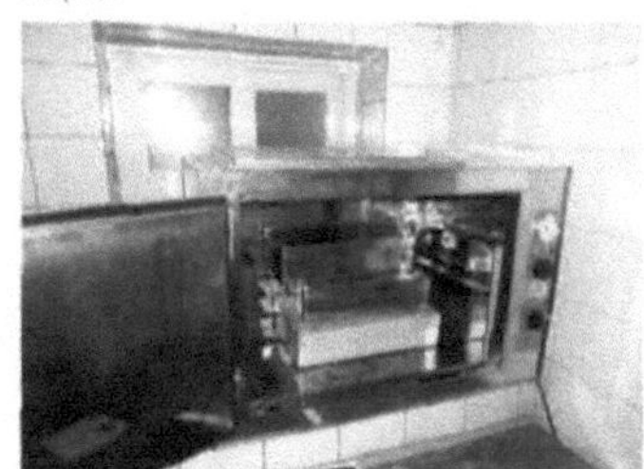

Stockage

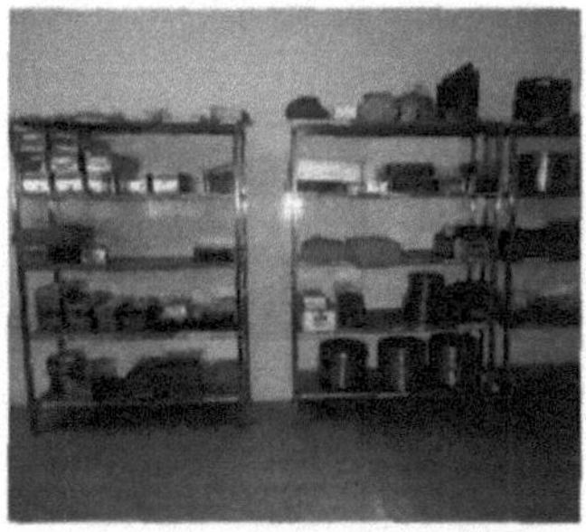

Stockage

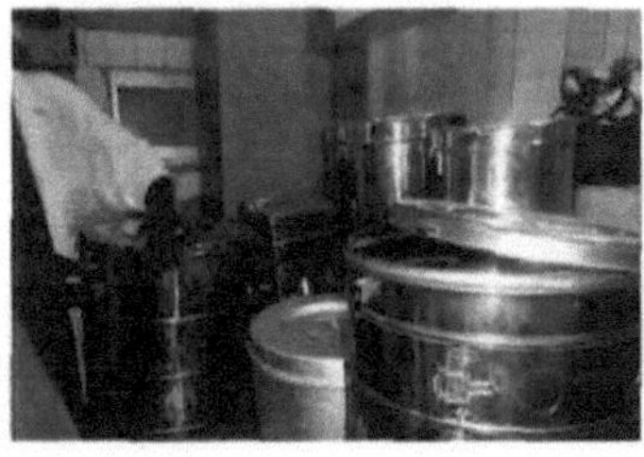

Surface (sol) de l'unité de stérilisation

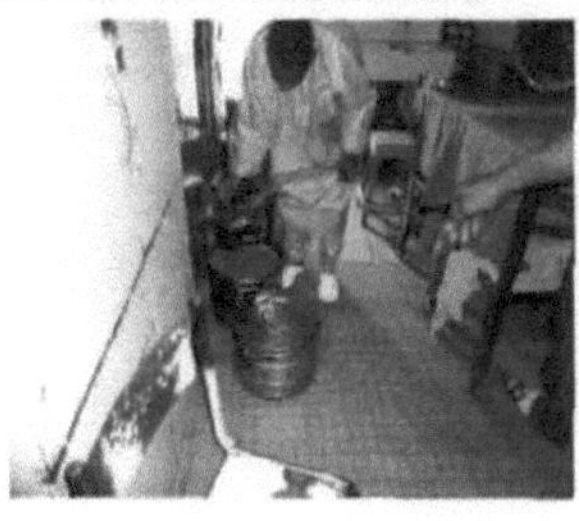

Surface (sol) de l'unité de stérilisation

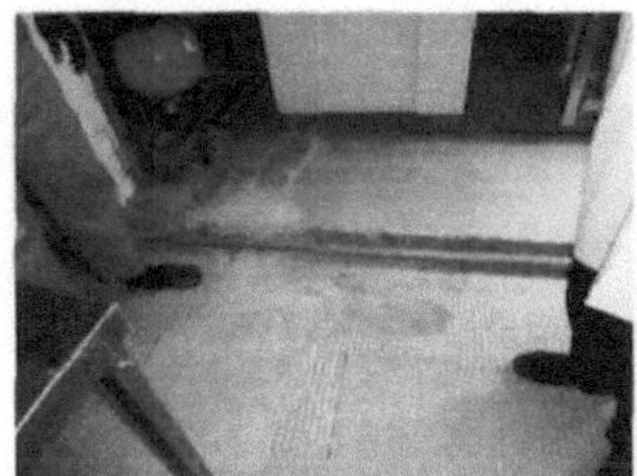